Fast & Tasty Meals for More Energy

Fast & Tasty Meals for More Energy

Written by Marieke Fourie.

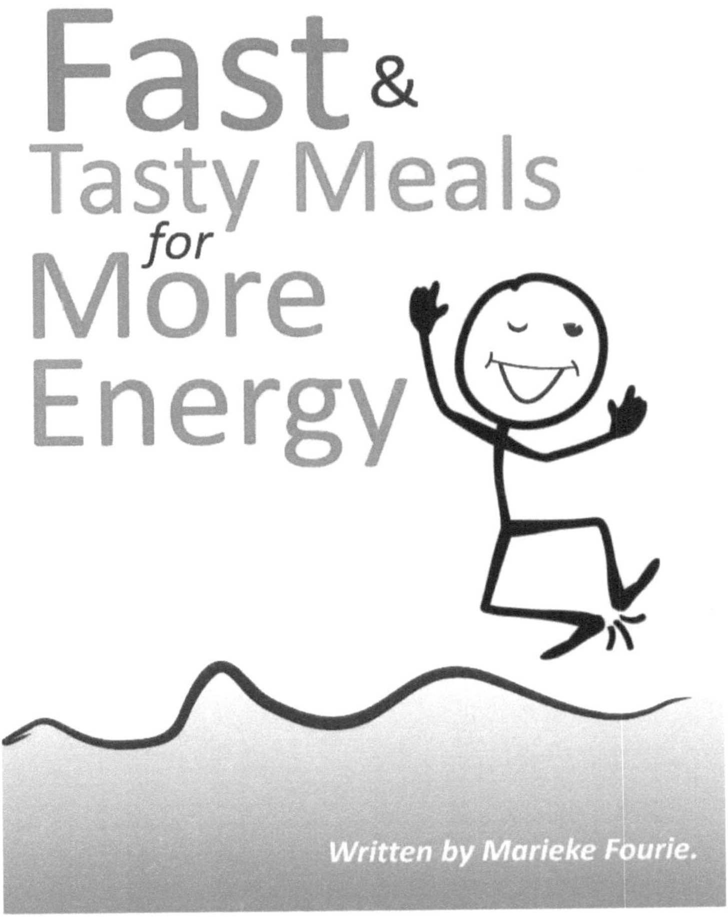

E-mail: creativity@ecofasteats.com

Facebook: https://www.facebook.com/ecofasteats/

Website: http://www.ecofasteats.com/

Other books: The Pumpkinskinman

ISBN: 9781539972624

Paeroa
2017

2

Contents

Introduction

I am interested in healthy living all my life. Although not always sticking to it!

Then I had to pay the price.....a headache or a nasty flu as a result of not eating sensibly.

Our hectic lifestyles need abundant energy.

I want to share my proven recipes for sustainable energy levels with you.

You will learn to make fast and easy meals yourself.

Eat as ecologically friendly as possible.

Learn to use what is available to you.

Be creative! You can do it!

Who am I and what is my body's needs?

In short, a human body needs;

- Vitamins and minerals, the mostly unknown essential ingredients that keep you going.
- Protein, the building blocks of your body.
- Fat, essential for your body's "telephone and computer" system, your brain and nerve cells.
- Fuel to keep you going. Choose the best fuel available.
- Water, all important water.

Do you know why you are feeling tired? Your body is telling you something, do you listen? Think about the food you eat.

- Where is it from?
- Is it good quality?
- What will this food do to my body?

- Why am I eating this?

Choose what is best for you. You deserve the best!

Prevent the midmorning and late afternoon tiredness by stable blood sugar levels.

- Why are blood glucose levels important?
- Why am I feelingbad?
- How do I know my blood glucose levels are low?

Bad food and good food. Choose the best quality available.

A quick fix I use when feeling low on energy.

Tiredness, iron and oxygen.

Haemoglobin, the oxygen carrier in your blood.

Some signs of too low iron levels in your body.

Foods with higher iron content.

Vitamin C and vitamin B, part of the iron carrier team.

Fat, the all-important coating of your telephone wires.

- Which oil is best to use?

The debate about good fat and bad fat is still going on. Decide for yourself.

Look at history and research statistics (or just eat different and evaluate yourself.)

Collect your own information.

Other uses for olive and coconut oils.

Water.

50 to 75% of your body consists of water.

Strokes, blood clots, kidney failure and more ailments caused by dehydration.

- How much water to I need?

Be aware who you are.

You are human.

You are smart. You can do your own research.

You can choose what to eat and drink.

- Why am I craving certain foods?
- What can I do about it?

You can be creative!

You will have heaps of energy to enjoy life!

Make every meal a celebration.

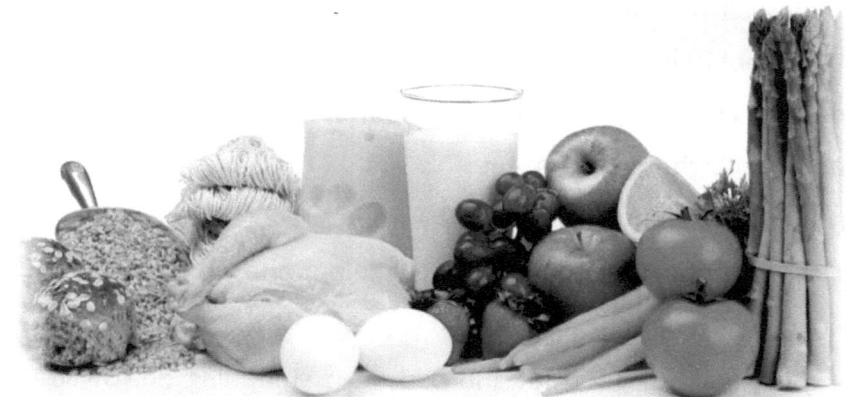

Chapter One: Introduction – Possible reasons for tiredness

I want to share my secret for endless energy with you! Understanding your body's food needs will help you to choose what is best for you.

Let me introduce myself. I am a nurse for 42 years, mostly for people at their workplace. I am a child of Africa, experienced to survive with scarce resources. These are proven recipes I share with you; I grew up on a farm with a sustainable lifestyle, my allergic child forced me to use only simple ingredients (no ready-made stuff from shops) and my circumstances taught me to make good meals with little money.

Our hectic lifestyles ask for abundant energy, yet we are often tired.

Possible reasons for your tiredness can be;

> - Unstable blood glucose levels (too much or too little sugar in your blood).
> - Dehydration (not enough water in your body)
> - Low iron levels.
> - Electrolyte imbalances (lack of essential nutrients).

The popular high sugar and caffeine drink for a "quick fix" helps only for a short time and it is NOT healthy. You will learn my secrets for fast, easy and tasty meals you can make yourself.

Tips to eat as ecologically friendly as possible;

➢ Grow your own ....even if it is only your own parsley and thyme in a pot. It is empowering to add your own fresh ingredients to your dishes, and super healthy.

➢ Learn to use what is available to you, be creative! The manufacturers and shops want you to believe ready- made, processed foods are best for you.

➢ Know that you are smart, if you learn to listen to your body and eat the foods you need, you will feel and look great!

Easy Eat Tip:

An on-the-run solution if you are in town and low on energy without food, is to buy;

➢ Pure orange juice, the natural sugars and minerals in orange juice works best for me.

➢ Banana, the potassium and natural sugars give you energy.

➢ A small packet of almonds to ensure your meal is more balanced with protein and oils as well.

This snack will keep your energy levels up till you have time for a proper meal.

Substitute the orange juice with any other pure juice or with milk (Amasi, sour milk, is actually better if you have a taste for it).

You can eat peanuts as second best in place of almonds. I often find most nuts other than almonds taste old and "moldy" when I buy it.

Chapter Two: Who am I and why do I need different foods?

I will only discuss some of the most important facts. If we compare our body to a car;

➢ Vitamins and minerals are like the small nuts and screws, keeping the wheels on and everything in place. The same as with a car, if you run short on these essential micro nutrients, your "wheels come off" Did you know your body only absorb calcium if boron is present as well as all the other role players?

➢ Protein is what the body is made of. Our bodies are been renewed all the time, if the building material is of poor quality, your body will have weak spots where "rust" can start.

➢ Fats and oils (lipids) is the "wiring" of your body, essential for your body's communication system (nerve cells). As with any electrical cord that needs insulation around, your body's "wires" are coated with lipids (fatty oil). If this coating around the nerve fibers gets bare patches with lipid cells missing, messages cannot pass smoothly. I witnessed several healthy individuals hospitalized with depression after a few months on a "fat free diet to lose weight".

➢ Energy to keep going, the fuel you need. Your body convert food to glucose, the energy every cell needs. Glucose that is not needed at that moment, is stored. As with most processes in the human body, the scientists are still researching to find out exactly how it all works. We do know not all foods are digested at the same speed and it is better to eat foods the body will take longer to convert into glucose.

➤ Water. Every living cell needs water. In the human body all processes need water.

Easy Eat Recipe

Warm Oats.

Yes, I know you get more vitamins if you eat the oats raw! But in winter it is cold and I want a hot breakfast! I believe to eat before I leave for work, but I will give you my easy recipe that you can do at home or at work.

Into a round plastic bowl with a lid

➤ 3 to 4 heaped desert spoons raw oats

➤ A pinch of salt

➤ About a teaspoon butter

➤ 1 teaspoon honey or about a desert spoon raisins

➤ A few almonds (if you want)

➤ Add a bit of milk till the oats are wet

When you want to eat at work, you just add boiling water till the consistency seems right, stirring vigorously while adding the water. Enjoy.

I personally do not feel safe to use a microwave, if you do use it to cook oats, turn it on medium power for two minutes as it will spill over and make a mess if cooking on high power.

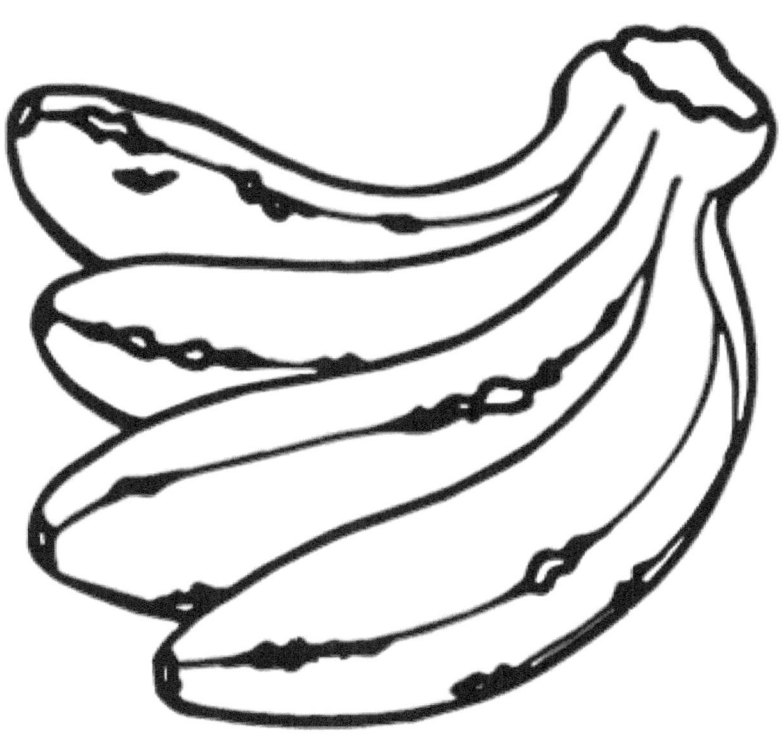

Chapter Three: Do you know why you are feeling tired?

Your body is talking, do you listen?

Think about the food you eat and what you drink. Where is this from? What are the ingredients? Is it good quality? Most governments have regulations for food safety, like the label on the packet must state the ingredients of the product. Do you read the label before you use the product? As example, do you know how bad for you Aspartame is?

What will this food do to my body? Can you see the vitamins in the apple handing out ammunition to your body's "army"? Can you see how fast your blood get the glucose energy balls to your brain after you drink the glass of water? Can you feel your muscles grow stronger after your good meal?

Why do I eat this? Is it good or maybe not good for me? Possible reasons for eating can be;

➤ body needs these nutrients,

➤ I am sad,

➤ I do not really want this but will eat to keep somebody else happy,

➤ I enjoy eating with my family?

If you stay aware why you eat and drink, it is easier to stick with good principles.

Be thankful for the food that is available to you.

Choose the best you can!

Most of the "manmade" foods give you a quick fix that push your blood sugar levels too high. The high blood sugar levels trigger your body's insulin alarm and lots of insulin are released. The sugar is processed fast and then too much insulin is running around in your system, causing the blood sugar level to drop too low. This "spiking" pattern of blood sugar levels makes you sick.

"High grade fuel" Foods…..the nearer the original source a food is, the better value for your body. Examples;

- ➤ Fresh sugar cane sticks, directly from the plants are full of vitamins and minerals.
- ➤ Nuts
- ➤ Pure fruit juice, water, carrot, celery sticks
- ➤ Dried fruit like raisins, peaches, etc.
- ➤ Apple, banana, other fruit, honey, whole wheat bread.

"Low grade fuel" Foods…the more machines a food go through, the lower value for your body. Examples;

- ➤ Potato crisps
- ➤ Soft drinks
- ➤ Donuts, cakes
- ➤ Sweets like toffees, lollipops, etc.

> Chips, burgers, foods fried in vegetable oil, sugar, white bread, etc.

Easy Eat Recipe

"Right around the kitchen" Stir fry.

A little boys' favourite food was when his mother looked in the cupboards and made a meal with what was available. I think it is a good name for a recipe!

Skin and cut 1 onion in rings.

Put your frying pan on the stove to heat, add about a teaspoon of coconut oil or olive oil. (I personally do not like to use butter for this….you can, if you prefer butter) Add the onions and stir frequently. About 3 minutes.

Wash and cut all the hard vegetables; potatoes, carrots, sweet potato, etc., in cubes, cut or peel off all the marks, "bad spots". If you are slow it is better to prepare everything before switching on the stove.

When onion rings are transparent and starting to get a golden colour, add the hard vegetables. Put on the lid. Turn down the heat a bit. Stir frequently. About 5 to 10 minutes.

Wash and cut the softer vegetables; broccoli, cabbage, mushrooms, etc., and add on top of your mix. Keep the heat on about 2 minutes more.

Switch off the heat.

Put the lid on and set your table. Stir.

Add salt and pepper if you want. I like a generous blob of sour cream or grated cheese on top when it is on my plate, especially when I do not have any meat with it.

Any left over chicken, fish, a tin of tuna, beef or meat cut up in pieces and added with the soft vegetables to heat up, add flavour and nutrition to your meal.

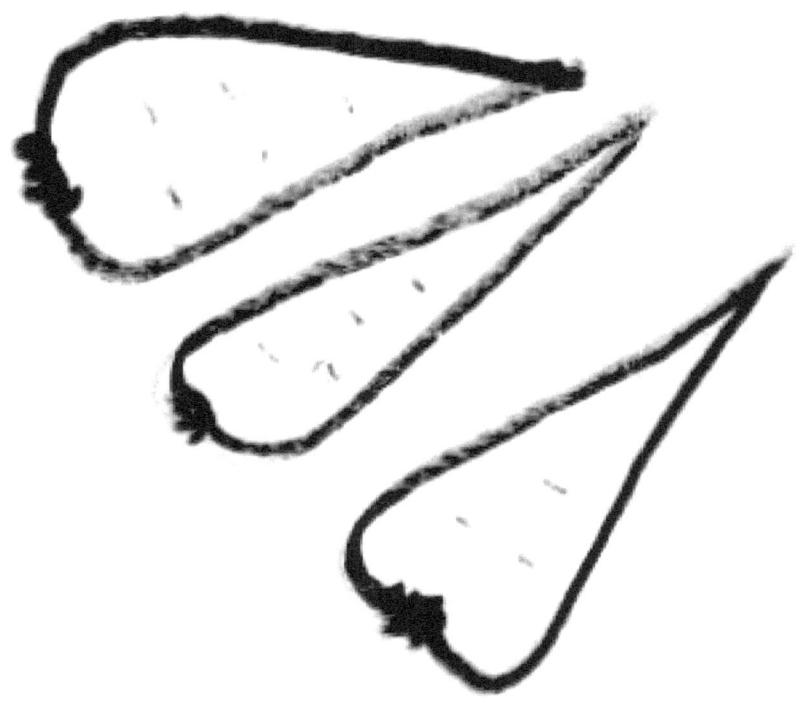

Chapter Four: Stabilize blood sugar levels.

Prevent mid-morning / late afternoon tiredness.

> ➢ Why are blood glucose levels important?

> ➢ Why do I feel bad in the mornings?

> ➢ How will I know if my blood glucose are too low?

Your blood sugar levels are very important as it measure if you have too much or too little glucose in your blood at that moment. A laboratory test can measure the glucose level inside your red blood cells. This test gives a median level of glucose in your bloodstream in the three months before your blood was taken.

Too low blood glucose levels put your body on high alert and your emergency systems kick in. If your body is unable to extract glucose from your body's stores (like in a diabetic with impaired sugar metabolism.........the emergency systems are not effective) you can get brain damage or even die within minutes. Keep your body's glucose "factory" healthy, eat good food!

Excessive alcohol use is dangerous as it damage your glucose "factory" and emergency response system.

There is some research about the good side of low blood sugar levels.

It is better to first ask your doctor if fasting will be good for you.

I agree with fasting at times. BUT you fast when you are at home, NOT at work. Low blood sugar levels make your risk for an accident much higher.

Choose to eat foods with good nutrients that will keep your blood sugar levels stable, not too high and not too low.

Some signs of low blood sugar; (Can you see these are risky around moving machines? Driving a car, is also operating a moving machine.)

- A "bad" quivering feeling in your gut, feeling anxious.
- Irritable.
- Angry.
- Dizzy.
- Headache.
- Weak feeling in your legs.

Tip; When I crave sweets or when my glucose levels are low, I rather eat a teaspoon of honey. It is better than refined sugar. Honey consists of two sugars; one is immediately available in your bloodstream, the second one is slow release.

- When the amount of glucose in the blood is too high it forms sharp crystals that cut and do permanent damage to the small blood vessels as in the eyes and kidneys.

➤ Most people are not aware when their blood glucose levels are too high. When the too high blood glucose is discovered with a medical examination, damage has already started.

➤ If the body's glucose mechanism is damaged, it is difficult to lead a normal life.

➤ You are smart! You can choose to eat good food and stay healthy!

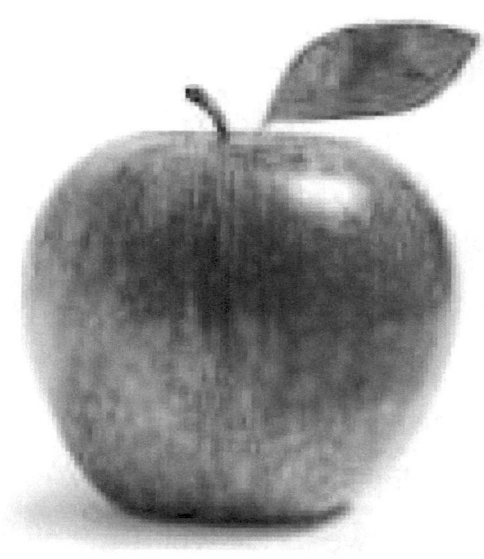

Chapter Five: Tiredness, Iron and Oxygen.

Iron is one of the micronutrients that is lacking in modern diets.

In my years of consulting ordinary men and women at work, I see a clear picture of iron deficiency in people who prefer take away fast foods.

How do I know if my tiredness is from low iron levels? ⏰
Some signs of anaemia (not enough iron in your blood)

- Irritable
- Emotional, cry easily
- Breathless feeling (as if a tight band is around your waist)
- Moody, feeling worthless
- Difficulty to sleep
- Yes! Low iron levels can present as depression.

Do you have enough iron in your blood to ensure adequate oxygen supply for optimum cell function?

Foods to boost your iron levels;

- Red meat
- Liver
- Eggs
- Green vegetables

- Beetroot
- Raisins

Your body needs Vitamin C and Vitamin B to be able to absorb iron, and the discovery around unknown micronutrients our bodies need, is ongoing.

If a person does not eat enough fruit and vegetables, the body cannot absorb the iron even if you eat enough eggs and red meat.

Easy Eat Recipe

Liver cakes

Ingredients

- About 1 cup minced liver (I prefer sheep liver)
- 1 egg
- 1 heaped desert spoon flour
- Salt and pepper
- 2 desert spoons vinegar
- Chopped and fried onions and tomato cubes (Optional)
- Add some parsley or mixed herbs if you want to.

Be creative!

How to

Fry the chopped onion in a heated frying pan with about a teaspoon of coconut oil or olive oil and add to your mix above.

Mix with spoon.

First, I bake one small bit to taste if I need to add more salt, pepper or vinegar.

With the spoon, put "blobs" of your mix into the frying pan. Remember to leave a little space for you to be able to turn your cakes over to be cooked on the other side.

Be careful to do this on medium heat. Rather bake it slower and make sure it is not pink on the inside any more.

Always do liver "well done" (completely cooked) as it is unsafe to eat raw liver because of possible germs and parasites. You should cook all meat products properly!

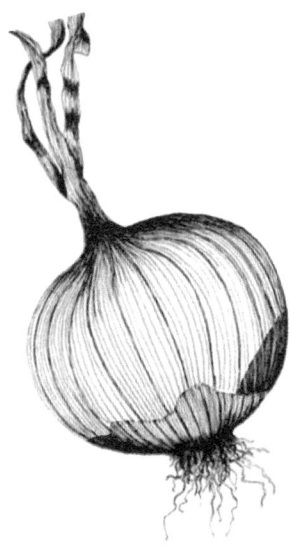

Chapter Six: Fat and oils, the all-important coating of your body's "telephone wires".

What is the best oil to use?

The debate about good fat and bad fat is still going on. Do your own research and decide for yourself. For the last 60 years we have been told only man made oils and spreads are good (like sunflower oil). Research that proved saturated "natural" fats are good, and best for you, was ignored. This controversy is still going on. You must decide for yourself.

I look at history

My mother is 96 years old, healthy and on no medication. She lived on a farm most of her life with homemade foods. I was in high school before I saw a bottle of sunflower oil for the first time.

I test it for myself

If I add a good scoop of sour cream or butter onto my eggs at breakfast, I do not need food till the evening meal. I witnessed several friends who substitute bread and sugar with saturated fats. They look and feel very good!

Easy Eat Recipe.

An omelette pancake, yes, it is both at once!

Into a bowl;

> ➤ 2 eggs

- ➢ About 20 ml milk
- ➢ Salt and pepper
- ➢ 1 heaped teaspoon self-raising flour (yes, easy wins mostly with me. I do use flour in my baking.) You can use almond flour or any flour you like or leave it altogether.
- ➢ I prefer a bit of coconut oil or sheep fat into a hot pan for my baking (you can use your preference.) I normally bake this mix in three batches. It looks like thick pancakes.

When one side is turning light brown, flip it over with an egg lifter to brown about 30 seconds on the other side as well.

Slide onto a heated plate.

Between the layers I will put what is available;

- ➢ Grated cheese with tomato cubes and fresh parsley.
- ➢ Or tuna
- ➢ Or cooked mince
- ➢ Anything you feel like.
- ➢ A blob of cream or butter on top will make sure you have enough fuel for the day.

This is a fast and easy way to feed unexpected visitors or hungry children from school.

For children I will maybe roll my pancake with the filling inside. This pancake around a banana is fast, fun, finger food.

You can be creative!

Tip

> ➤ I often use coconut oil to revive my skin as well. It works as a cleanser as well as a moisturiser.

> ➤ For thousands of years, up to today, olive oil is used to keep babies' and old people's skins' soft and supple.

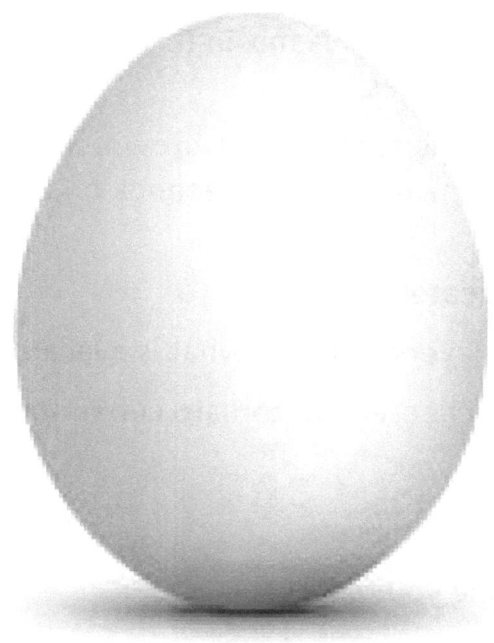

Chapter Seven: Water – How much do I need

50% to 75% of your body is water.

> ➢ Every living cell needs water.
> ➢ Blood clots, strokes and kidney failure are some of the ailments caused by not drinking enough water.

How much water do I need? Tips to help you drink more water.

Experiment with your own mixes;

Add half a sliced lemon and the same amount of cucumber slices to a litre of tap water, refrigerate if you prefer and drink from that as often as you like.

Add a dash of lemon juice or apple cider vinegar to your water, you can add a spoon of honey and/ or a twig of Rosemary, a peppermint leave, etc.

Be creative! Make your own good tasting beverages with just water and spices, like a cinnamon stick into boiled water with honey.

As it is winter where I am at the moment, I just add boiled water to a slice of lemon for a hot drink, sometimes with a teaspoon of honey stirred in as well.

Remember to first boil the water and let it cool down before use, if you are in an area with unsafe drinking water!

Chapter Eight: Be aware who you are.

You are human. You will have heaps of energy to enjoy life if you fulfil your body's needs. You can choose what to eat and drink. Choose the best you can!

You will have your body with you till you die. Do you really need this too expensive smart car/clothes/house that you will only enjoy for a short while? Do not spend all your money on temporary luxuries.

Never ever compromise on the quality of your food!

Make every meal a celebration, say thank you for what you have. It is a good tradition for the family to eat at least one meal a day around a table, talking to each other. Pick an interesting subject all can participate in.

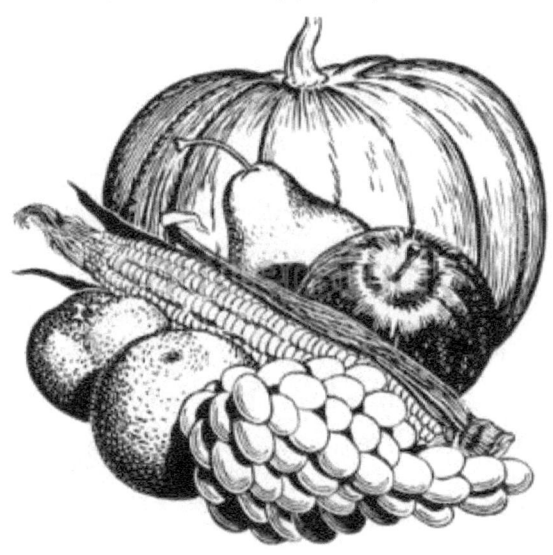

Recipes

Meat balls.

- ➤ 1 heaped desert spoon raw oats (I prefer the finer oats)
- ➤ 3 desert spoons vinegar
- ➤ ½ teaspoon salt
- ➤ A pinch pepper
- ➤ 1 egg
- ➤ A squirt of Worcestershire sauce

You can add

- ➤ 1 finely chopped onion
- ➤ Grated carrot, grated courgette, grated potato and grated sweet potato.

NOTE: If you add a lot of vegetables, it is wise to add more herbs and spices and seasoning. I often add cloves, ginger, mixed herbs, parsley, tomato cubes, chilli crumbs.

To Make:

Mix well together and roll balls in the size you want.

Pack the balls, NOT on top of each other, in a saucepan, with a little oil.

 Saucepan onto the stove top on medium heat. When it starts to sizzle, add about 3mm water and put the lid on.

Check regularly. Cook until the meat- balls get a nice

brown crust at the bottom......this can be tricky to achieve. Sometimes it is easier to put it in the oven under the grill for two to three minutes to get a crispy finish.

If I am in a hurry, (I normally am!) I will add little cubes of fresh vegetables or some frozen vegetables on top and not bother too much about browning.

To improve the taste and the looks of my dish I sometimes add tomato paste, curry powder and beef stock powder and thicken the sauce for a meatballs and gravy dish.

I use this basic recipe for fried hamburger patties as well. Just put a little oil into a heated pan and fry about 3 minutes each side till cooked.

You can substitute the meat with chicken or fish (then rather use lemon juice to replace vinegar) or use cooked and mashed lentils or dried beans.

Sauce Tips

▶ Put a heaped spoon of gravy powder, the variety that thickens, into a mug.

▶ Add a little bit of cold water and mix to a slobbery paste

▶ Add boiling water while you stir vigorously with a fork (sauce is now half cooked)

▶ Add to your still boiling dish and stir.

When I do not want to upset my arrangement in my pot, instead of stirring, I pick up the pot and tilt it from side to side to mix the sauce with the liquids in the pot.

To make the sauce more interesting; add a dash of tomato paste, curry powder, Worcestershire sauce, chutney or mixed herbs when mixing stock powder and cold water.

Another fast fix when the liquids in your dish are not thick and interesting enough:

Use "Cup of Soup". I turn the heat off and then tilt the pot to get a little "dam" of liquid in one place. Add the soup powder and stir with a fork till mixed, then tilt the pot from side to side to mix it through with the rest of the liquids in the pot.

You can use any instant soup this way.

The flavours I mostly use are "Mushroom" or "Tomato".

Lentils and rice

Cook lentils and rice together, if you use rice that takes longer to cook, (some varieties cook faster) add the lentils about two minutes after the rice starts to cook to make sure all is done at the same time.

To Make:

▶ In a saucepan, add boiling water to the rice and lentils till the water level is 2cm above the dry ingredients.

▶ Cook on stove top on medium heat without lid on saucepan for about 15 minutes.

▶ I prefer to add and stir salt through, just before the last bit of water evaporates.

▶ I find it unnecessary to drain water off rice or lentils

if you stick to the right amount of water from the start.

▶ Sprinkle with pepper and/or mixed herbs. Serve hot as a protein-rich side dish with any saucy main dish like a casserole or butter chicken.

Lentil salad

As the main ingredient, use the cooled down left-overs from the above recipe, or cook a fresh batch with only lentils. Lentils cook quickly, about 15 minutes. If after they are cooked there is still too much water, you will have to drain off the excess.

When cooled, add:

▶ Chopped onion

▶ Mixed herbs

▶ Small cubes of fresh or dried tomato

▶ Pepper

▶ Frozen peas

▶ Fresh or pickled cucumber

As salad dressing use cottage cheese or plain yogurt or sour cream or mayonnaise or whatever you like.

This is a good meal to take to work, especially if you add the frozen peas in the morning, by lunchtime your salad will still be cold.

Spinach, hot or cold iron booster

Fill the sink with clean, cold water and submerge a bunch of spinach in the water.

Put your pot with 1cm of water on the stove on medium heat.

Peel and cut 1 onion in rings and add to the water as it start boiling. Cook with lid on.

Scrub and cube 2 medium potatoes or sweet potato and add.

Start to rinse and clean the spinach leaves one by one. If too sandy, use running water. I do not use a knife any more to cut the stems off, I just grab the stem in one hand, and with my other hand I tear off the leafy parts. All the cleaned and separated leaves go into a large bowl. When finished (this takes about 5 minutes), the onion and potato are partly cooked. Add spinach leaves on top of them. Check that there is at least 2mm of water left in the pot and put the lid on.

In about 5 minutes the spinach should be cooked. Switch off the heat.

Take the pot off the stove and place on a stable heat-proof workspace and mash onion, potato/sweet potato and spinach together in the pot.

I add my butter/coconut oil/sheep fat/lard or olive oil at this stage to let it melt.

After cooled down till about body temperature; add the rest of your ingredients.

> ➢ Salt and pepper to taste

> ➢ 1 heaped desert spoon flour (I prefer self-raising flour) You can use almond flour or just add more potato.

> ➢ 1 egg

Mix well and scoop into a flat pie dish, smooth it on top.

Sprinkle grated cheese on top and/or garnish with a few strips of streaky bacon.

Bake in a medium oven for about 40 minutes.

If you serve this straight from the oven, it tends to be a bit wobbly. Best to let it cool off a bit.

Served cold, cut in wedges, I's great to pack in a lunchbox.

Mince with hidden vegetables.

It is often a challenge to keep family meals balanced. Here is my secret for fantastic mince!

Peel and cut 1 onion into rings. Onions boost your immunity!

Put onion into saucepan on stove and switch heat on. No fat or oil is needed.

The moment when the onion starts to sizzle and get brown, add the mince. Stir with a fork.

The smell when meat starts to cook can be a bit strong so, to combat the odour, add salt and a squirt of lemon juice or vinegar (not too much as your meal can be too sour)

Stir frequently and let mince and onions brown…..if it has not enough fat, it will burn easily. Add oil or fat or if you want to cut on fats/oils, add a bit of water.

At the same time, wash and grate vegetables. Potato, sweet potato, carrot, georgettes, cabbage. Add on top of browned mince and onion. The vegetables should be about two thirds and the mince one third. Do not stir. Put the lid on.

Add about two spoons of tomato paste and/or a can of tinned tomatoes. (I like to use lots of red stuff to camouflage the carrot) Do not stir. Turn heat down. Keep lid on. Cook for 15 to 20 minutes.

I like to add chutney in the end……as alternative I add 2 to 3 dried apricots or peaches with the vegetables to give enough time for the fruit to soften.

Take the pot off the stove and place on a safe heat-proof workspace and mash all together.

Add more salt if needed, add pepper, cloves, nutmeg, ginger, small slivers of chilies and peppers, mustard, mushrooms, a squirt of Worcestershire sauce, a blob of chutney or apricot jam, ¼ teaspoon Marmite or Vegemite. Experiment, add and omit as you please.

Taste and add till you are happy……if it is maybe still a bit too watery, thicken with gravy powder or part of a packet of brown onion soup.

► To make your meal more attractive, scoop it onto pancakes or into a baking dish as a pie.

► Be creative with a topping to cover the mince! Try cooked and mashed cauliflower with butter......sprinkle cheese on top and grill for 5 to 10 minutes till golden brown.

Or mix together:

► 1 desert spoon oil, or melted coconut oil or butter

► Salt and pepper

► 2 heaped desert spoons self-raising flour

► Add water till it is like a thick custard.

► Put blobs of this dough all over the mince mix to cover all.....you can sprinkle a bit of grated cheese on top if you want.

► Bake on high heat for about 20 minutes till golden brown.

Or

► Cook potatoes or sweet potatoes or both (combined it taste marvelous!) in water till soft.

► Mash together with butter and salt added.

► Use as topping with your mince.

Or

► Use in lasagna or with cooked spaghetti.

Half hour soup.

Ingredients

▶ 4 potatoes or sweet potatoes (I prefer sweet potatoes) peeled

▶ 1 kg carrots peeled

Cook the above in water on the stove. I do not use too much water, I find it cooks faster with less water. Keep the lid on.

▶ 1 tin of tomatoes, add when the vegetables are soft.

I roughly cut the vegetables in 4 pieces each before cooking, normally they are soft after about 20 minutes.

If you want to be really fast, cut the vegetables in smaller cubes. When vegetables are soft, mash it in the pot.

Add boiling water to thin.

Add one packet of Minestrone soup and cook another 5 minutes. See tip below.

Add salt and pepper to taste and serve.

Add a generous blob of sour cream in the middle of each soup serving. (Optional)

You can add to this recipe, I like to add meat casserole leftovers or a few sausages.

Tip

When you want to add thickener to a boiling pot, do it the other way around; mix the soup powder with a bit of cold water in a container with a volume of at least 500ml.

Then, using a soup ladle, add some of the boiling mix to the soup powder mix and stir vigorously.

Add to the boiling pot and stir.

This way around clots do not form easily.

Rinse the soup powder mix container with a bit of water and add to your pot

Broccoli and Feta cheese

Broccoli is a wonderful vegetable. If picked fresh from your garden, it taste sweeter and is tasty to use raw in salads. It is really very easy to grow. Put a few plants in a pot if you do not have a garden.

From one head, put only broccoli florets, volume about two cups, into boiling water for 1 minute, drain water off.

(Keep the broccoli stems to add to soup or stews.)

Arrange broccoli in a flat baking dish.

Crumble feta cheese into the spaces between broccoli florets.

Mix into another bowl;

> ➤ 2 eggs
> ➤ 1 heaped desert spoon flour
> ➤ Salt and pepper
> ➤ ½ teaspoon of dried mixed herbs
> ➤ ½ cup milk
> ➤ 1 desert spoon cream or sour cream.

Pour the egg mix over the broccoli. Make sure to put some over every floret.

Sprinkle grated cheese on top and bake in the oven on medium heat for 30 to 40 minutes till cooked.

Grind some black pepper on top.

As a variation, and faster as well, toss the blanched broccoli with some seedless raisins, nuts and small cheese cubes (or feta cheese) together in a bowl. Add seasoning and/or salad dressing to taste.

Another variation

Cook 1.5cm sweet potato cubes in 3mm of water for 3 minutes.

Add broccoli florets and stems also cut in the same size cubes and cook 1 minute more.

That's it! A fast and tasty side dish to add to your filled pancakes or what you have.

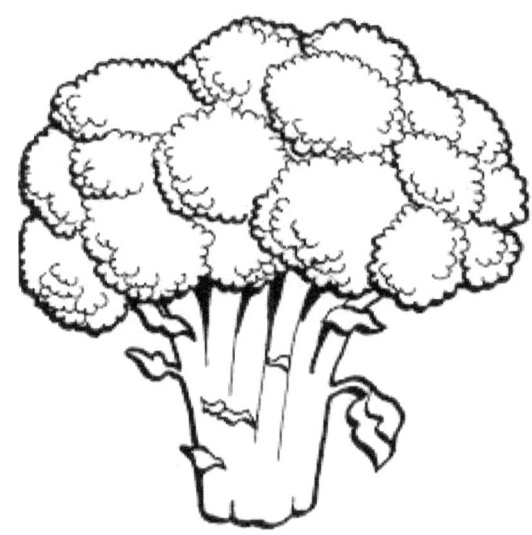

Pumpkin

It can be difficult to skin pumpkin when the skin is hard.

When the skin is softer and you do skin it, use the peel to cut little manikins if you are lucky enough to have small children around.

I cut it about 8cm long, with a head, two arms and two legs. Use the sharp point of your knife to mark two eyes and a smile. Enjoy the fun!

I do not skin pumpkin any more (see below).

Easy cooking tips.

Wash the pumpkin properly. Cut it in halves or quarters. Remove the seeds with a spoon. Pack the pumpkin pieces into a large enough pot, add water, put the lid on, and cook till soft. Depending on the size, it takes half an hour or longer.

▶ Use just enough water to finish cooking the pumpkin. You do not want to throw away vitamins and minerals with excessive water.

Remove from heat when cooked and let it cool down enough to enable you to peel off the outer skin. I use a knife and fork and help with my fingers to grab the papery skin.

▶ I prefer to leave the green layer as it contains important nutrients.

With this base of pumpkin (I mash it to a smooth texture) you can create different dishes.

Pumpkin variations

Use it with salt and pepper as a base or topping for meat, chicken or fish dishes.

Mix with sweet potato, potato, lentils and peas (add or leave ingredients as you wish), an egg, some grated cheese, butter, a bit of flour and bake in an oven for a meat-free dish.

For the ones who like a bit of sweet stuff, read on.

Sweet Pumpkin Tart

I never bake messy, oily, time consuming little cakes on the stove top any more. This is much easier and tasty as well.

Into about 2 cups of the cooked pumpkin mash, add:

1 desert spoon butter or coconut oil

¼ cup brown sugar, xylitol, stevia or any other natural sweetener

1 egg (Add the egg and flour when pumpkin is cooled down to at least body temperature, otherwise the egg will cook as you put it in.)

2 heaped desert spoons wheat flour; almond flour or any flour you like. If the cooked tart is too "wobbly", increase the amount of flour to suit, or put your mix in a pie crust (American Style)

¼ to ½ teaspoon of ground cinnamon

Mix all together and spoon into an oven dish. Flatten on

top.

Bake with medium heat, 150 to 180 degrees Celsius till light brown on top and cooked through.

Let it cool down a bit before cutting and serving.

I often serve this cold as well, cut into 5cm blocks.

This blocks of pumpkin tart freeze well.

I freeze it packed like a puzzle in a plastic bag, break off as many pieces as needed, thaw and heat it for an instant side dish.

Easy potato bake

Peel and wash 4 potatoes, cut in 3mm discs or 1 cm cubes.

Arrange evenly into an oven dish.

Mix together; 300ml of fresh cream or milk and a packet of white onion soup or mushroom soup or cream/milk with salt, pepper and mixed herbs added.

Pour this mix over the potatoes, sprinkle grated cheese on top and bake for about one hour in a medium hot oven till potatoes are soft.

If you use milk, it is best with a few bits of butter sprinkled on top.

You can also add bacon pieces.

Stove top potato dish

Skin and cut 1 onion in rings.

Add 1 teaspoon of coconut/olive oil to a heated saucepan.

Add onion rings, turn heat down a bit and stir.

While the onion rings are on the heat, wash and cube 2 to 3 potatoes. (If the skins are marked too much or if you prefer, peel and cube).

When the onion are starting to brown, add the potato cubes and put the lid on.

Stir frequently. Add a bit more oil or a teaspoon of water at a time to prevent your dish burning.

The potatoes should be soft and cooked but still in shape. It takes about 5 to 10 minutes to cook.

Add salt and pepper to taste and serve as side dish.

Butter chicken

Put 1 Onion, cut into rings, into a heated saucepan with oil.

Add 500gm chicken pieces and stir.

When the above is browned, add:

2 desert spoons tomato paste

Salt and pepper

¼ teaspoon curry powder, or to your taste

½ teaspoon turmeric

A dash of ground ginger or ½ teaspoon of fresh ginger cut in small pieces.

Add 150ml of apricot yogurt.

Put the lid on and simmer on low heat till cooked.

Add fresh beans and/or carrot pieces and/or frozen peas about two minutes before taking off heat.

Optionally you can add:

➢ 100ml fresh cream or sour cream (if you use sour cream, add a spoon of chutney as well.)

➢ Any herbs or spices you like.

Easy Chicken dish

Put 3 chicken breasts into a saucepan with 1 large onion cut into rings.

Cook on low heat with the lid on till tender. Takes 20 to 30 minutes.

With a knife and fork, remove all bones and cut the chicken sideways into 1cm pieces.

Add water till total liquid is about 400ml.

Add mushrooms and any other vegetables you like.

Add a packet of white onion soup or mushroom soup and cook 5 minutes longer. It is then ready to serve.

You can use the above mix as the filling for a chicken pie.

Tuna and pasta

You can use any pasta you like, I prefer pasta shells. Maybe you prefer gluten free rice pasta.

Put 2 cups dried pasta into a pot and add salt, pepper and a blob of butter or a teaspoon of oil.

Add boiling water till it is 2cm above pasta, stir and cook without a lid on.

Cook pasta for 10 minutes till soft. Drain excess water.

Start white sauce while pasta is cooking;

> ➢ 500ml milk into a pot on the stove

> ➢ Mix corn flour with a bit of cold water, remember to use a 1litre container as you will add the boiling milk to the cold mix. Follow the instructions on the packet and use the amount for a thick sauce.

NOTE: It is best to stir with a whisk when you add the boiling milk to corn flour mix. While you can use wheat flour, I prefer corn flour. When the corn flour and hot milk are mixed, return the mixture to the pot on the stove and stir till evenly thickened.

When white sauce is cooked, add to pasta in pot.

Add one tin of tuna.

Add salt and pepper to taste

Mix together and serve while hot with a sprinkling of cheese on top.

NOTE: Many recipes put this mix into an oven dish and

bake it with cheese on top.....I stopped doing that. Rather, make it more interesting by grinding black pepper on top and/or add a sprinkling of dried or fresh herbs.

Basic fish cakes

I grew up with this recipe. It was one of the few "shop" foods we ate.

Mix together:

- ➢ 1 tin Tomato pilchards
- ➢ 1 egg
- ➢ Salt and pepper
- ➢ 1 heaped desert spoon self-raising flour.

Add coconut oil, lard or oil of your choice to a heated pan on the stovetop. With a dessert spoon put blobs of the above mix into the heated pan. Leave about 2 cm spaces between the blobs as the cakes increase in size.

Note: Remember to turn the heat on medium....if it is too hot, your food will burn on the outside and not cook in the middle. Turn over with a spatula or "egg lifter".

About 3 minutes on each side should give you a nice golden brown colour on the outside.

I always break the biggest one in the middle to check if it is properly cooked.......and taste your first batch to see if you must add maybe more salt.

Try to add parsley snippets as a variation, or maybe chopped onion.

Serve warm with homemade bread or with mash.

Cold fish cakes with some sandwiches or salad do well for a lunch box.

Dried bean soup

Empty a 500gm packet of dried beans onto a clean workspace.

Working from the part nearest to you, remove all possible damaged beans or other debris. Slide the clean beans into a pot, or into a colander if you see sand you need to wash off before cooking.

Rinse beans with cold water.

Most recipes let you soak the beans overnight. I skip this step.

Cover beans in the pot with cold water; level about 5 cm above beans.

I prefer to add some meaty bones to the beans. Mutton or beef shin is great.

With lid on pot, put stove on medium to high heat.

When it starts to cook, turn the heat down to very, very slow. Or, if you want to save electricity, you put the stove off and transfer the boiling pot to your energy saver box for 4 to 12 hours. See about energy saver cooking below.

Your soup pot must cook very slowly, so that you do not have messy spilling over, and it is less likely to burn in the bottom of the pot.

Check the water level and stir about every half hour, if the beans become exposed, add some boiling water.

After about two hours, add other vegetables like onion, carrots if you want. Stir. Check if the beans become soft.

When the beans are soft, and can be easily crushed with your stirring spoon, add salt, pepper, herbs, dash of lemon juice or vinegar and a dash of Worcestershire sauce.

Some like to use a blender to make a smooth soup. I prefer it as it is, as most of the beans will be falling apart. Soft and mulchy.

If you find the soup is too watery, you can add a handful of raw oats and cook 5 minutes longer, or mix a packet of soup powder with a bit of cold water and add to thicken.

This is a large quantity. It freezes well for future use.

Tip

Never add salt to raw, dried legumes (beans, peas, etc.) The salt prevents the beans to cook soft. After hours of cooking, the beans will still be hard.

Pea soup

Do as for the dried bean soup, with some differences:

Substitute split peas for the beans.

As the peas cook much faster, the soup can be ready within two hours.

Peas will burn easily at the bottom.

> ➢ Stove heat must be very low.

> ➢ Stir regularly with a wooden spoon.

> ➤ Do not leave on the heat after peas are cooked and mushy.

Peas are a pest for boiling over, so cook with the lid askew or with the lid off altogether.

Tip: Energy saving "Slow cooker"

An electrical slow cooker is good to use, but I prefer this method:

The principle is to prevent the heat from escaping the cooking pot.

Use what is available to you in your area. If you live in a grain producing area, you will have straw. If you live in a city, you have newspapers.

Take a box, about 4 times the size of your pot.

Line all sides and the bottom with newspapers, layer upon layer. Then crumple single newspaper pages to make "insulation balls".

When the meat is cooked through (no longer raw), put the still boiling pot with lid on, into the box and quickly stuff all open areas around the pot with the insulation balls.

On top of the pot put more newspapers and cover.

The idea is that no heat must be able to escape from the pot.

If you use straw, just make sure it is tightly packed all around and on top.

You may be able to buy different "cook boxes" from local suppliers. I prefer to make my own.

My mother had a special blanket that she used to keep the dough warm when she was making bread.

When you are ready to finish cooking the soup, take out the pot from the box. It should be almost soft and will need less time on the stove.

PLEASE NOTE: Be careful not to leave food longer than 10 hours in the box and *always cook it again before eating*.

Easy, Tasty Bread

Making your own bread was normal 100 years ago. Why not today? If you love bread, try to make your own.

You can look up a recipe or use the one on the flour packet.

I take shortcuts;

Boil the kettle.

Spray the bread pan with a non-stick spray (if you do not have non-stick pans) You can also use a muffin pan. I often wash and use tuna tins.

Put a heaped desert spoon of butter or coconut oil into a jug. Pour about 200ml boiling water over. As alternative you can use olive oil, or no fat at all.

When the butter or oil is liquid, add 200ml cold water to the jug with the oil to make up 400ml liquid, making the water a bit warmer than body temperature. The temperature of this water is important; if it is too hot it will kill the yeast, if it is too cold the bread will not rise.

Into a large bowl add:

> ➢ 500gm brown bread or whole wheat flour
>
> ➢ 1 teaspoon fine salt
>
> ➢ ½ teaspoon sugar (to help the yeast along faster)
>
> ➢ 1 sachet of dried yeast granules (I use 8gm sachets)
>
> ➢ As variation add any or all of these; raisins, date pieces, almonds, pumpkin seeds, mixed herbs, cinnamon, ginger, etc. Mix these with the dry ingredients.

Before you start to mix and get your hands all messy.......switch the oven on 50 degrees Celsius (just warmer than body temperature) and make sure everything is ready around you. It is handy to keep the flour packet still there, and to have more lukewarm water nearby.

Pour the oil/fat and water mix into bowl with dry ingredients and mix thoroughly. Add water or a bit of flour to get the right consistency. If you mix the dough well enough it will become less sticky and you can form it onto an oblong shape to put into the pan. I still struggle (after 40 years) to get my bread as smart as Mum's!

Do not worry about it. I tend to add too much liquid to my bread, resulting in a flattened top when baked. It still tastes way better than the shop's bread!

Fill the pan only two thirds of the volume capacity.

Wet your hands and smooth the top of the dough.

Put the pan into the slightly warm oven.

After 5 minutes check if it is not too warm in the oven. If it is too hot to touch, switch off the oven.

After 20 to 30 minutes when the pan is full, switch the oven on 200 degrees Celsius.

Rather put the pan on the lower shelf. It can be tricky if you see your bread is burning on the top as your bread will collapse if you open the oven door during baking.

When you smell the bread and it has shrunk away from the sides of the pan, it is ready. Baking time is about 45 minutes.

Switch off the oven and remove the pan with oven gloves.

Turn the pan upside down onto a cooling rack and the bread will slide out.

Let it cool a bit before cutting. Enjoy!

Beetroot tips

Buy young beetroot, (the smaller ones) if you prefer to eat it without sauces, as they are softer and sweeter.

Always buy firm, fresh vegetables and fruit.

If the leaves are fresh and in good condition, you can use them as well; raw in salads or cooked with other vegetables.

Before cooking, take off the leaves.

Put the beetroot in a large pot. Cover completely with cold

water, making sure that two thirds of the pot is still empty.

Start cooking on medium heat with the lid askew and when it start to cook, turn the heat right down. I would rather cook beetroot longer, about one hour on low heat, than clean up all that red spluttering mess on the stove and everywhere!

When beetroot is cooked…..soft when you prick it with a fork, turn off the heat.

Empty the boiling water from the pot and fill it halfway with cold water. Leave the pot in the sink to avoid messing on your work surface.

If you grab a beetroot with your hand, the skin should come right off. Use a knife to trim the top and bottom bits if needed and transfer the cleaned ones to a bowl.

When the water in the pot becomes too warm, drain some off and add more cold water.

When you are finished skinning the beetroots, the beetroot peels with the water in the pot are easy to clear away. Just throw them into your garden compost.

Using this method you will have very little cleaning to do.

Remember, life is too short to waste time feeling bad.

Discover your creative side.

Eat good food and enjoy lots of energy.

May Good Health and Bountiful Energy be your constant companions.

Marieke.